DYLAN PULSE

Nutrition for Active Seniors

Short Guide to Unlocking Longevity Diet Secrets for Elderly Fitness and Energy Boosting Even if You Think You're Too Old to Start

This book was professionally typeset on Reedsy.
Find out more at reedsy.com

Contents

1 Introduction 1

2 Understanding Nutritional Needs of Active Seniors 3

3 Special Nutritional Considerations for Seniors 8

4 Meal Planning and Preparation 19

5 Supplements for Active Seniors 45

6 Staying Motivated and Making Informed Choices 53

7 Conclusion 58

8 References 60

1

Introduction

Welcome to a guide confronting the conventional wisdom about aging and nutrition head-on. It's crafted for those of you who, despite advancing years, are not willing to settle for a passive approach to health. This book is a practical toolkit for active seniors determined to maintain and enhance their vitality, energy, and overall quality of life through informed dietary choices.

Here, complexity gives way to clarity. This book simplifies nutritional guidelines, making them accessible and actionable. It is not just talking theory; it provides simple, budget-friendly recipes that consider dietary needs and the physical and financial realities you might face.

But this book goes beyond mere meal plans. It's a resource for tackling common health challenges such as diabetes and hypertension through dietary adjustments. The aim is to offer solutions and sustainable strategies that fit your lifestyle and help you manage health conditions more effectively.

Expect to find:

- Clear, straightforward advice on nutrition for seniors, cutting through the scientific jargon.
- Practical, easy-to-prepare recipes designed with senior-specific nutritional needs in mind.
- Tips for meal planning and preparation that respect your time, budget, and physical capabilities.
- Strategies for staying motivated and making informed food choices that can improve health and energy levels.

You're in the right place if you want to transform your dietary habits to support a more active, healthful lifestyle. This book is your stepping stone to a richer, fuller experience in your senior years, proving that it's always possible to make changes that can significantly enhance your well-being.

2

Understanding Nutritional Needs of Active Seniors

Macronutrients: Proteins, Carbohydrates, Fats

Macronutrients are the cornerstone of any diet, providing the energy and building blocks our bodies need to function optimally. For active seniors, understanding and managing the intake of these nutrients is essential for maintaining muscle mass, ensuring energy levels, and supporting overall health.

Proteins: Proteins are crucial for repairing and building tissues, including muscles, which is especially important for seniors engaged in any form of physical activity. The recommended daily intake (RDI) for seniors is higher than for younger adults to prevent muscle loss associated with aging. A guideline is 1.0 to 1.2 grams of protein per kilogram of body weight. For a senior weighing 70 kg (about 154 lbs), this means at least 70 to 84 grams of protein daily. Best sources include:

- Lean meats (chicken, turkey, beef)

- Fish (especially fatty fish like salmon, which also provides omega-3 fatty acids)
- Dairy products (milk, yogurt, cheese)
- Plant-based proteins (legumes, lentils, chickpeas, tofu, quinoa)

Carbohydrates: Carbohydrates are the primary energy source for the body. They're essential for fueling regular physical activity. Complex carbohydrates, with their high fiber content, are preferred for their slower digestion and more stable blood sugar levels. The general recommendation for carbohydrate intake is about 45-65% of total daily calories. For an active senior consuming 2,000 calories daily, this translates to 225-325 grams of carbohydrates daily. Best sources include:

- Whole grains (brown rice, oats, whole wheat bread)
- Vegetables (especially leafy greens)
- Fruits (berries, apples, bananas)
- Legumes (beans, lentils)

Fats: Fats are essential for nutrient absorption, brain health, and energy. However, the focus should be on healthy fats. The RDI for fats is about 20-35% of total daily calories, focusing on unsaturated fats. A 2,000-calorie diet means 44-78 grams of fat per day. Best sources include:

- Unsaturated fats (olive oil, avocado, nuts, seeds)
- Omega-3 fatty acids (fatty fish like salmon, mackerel, and sardines; flaxseeds, walnuts)

For active seniors, balancing these macronutrients with physical activity levels and health goals is critical to supporting a vibrant, healthy lifestyle. Ensuring a diet rich in these nutrients can help maintain muscle mass, provide energy for activities, and support overall well-being.

Micronutrients: Vitamins and Minerals

Micronutrients support the body's functions, from bone health and energy metabolism to immune system performance. Active seniors need to focus on getting adequate vitamins and minerals to support their increased activity levels and physiological needs.

For Bone Health:

- **Calcium:** Fundamental for bone strength and density. The recommended daily intake for seniors is 1,200 mg. Sources include dairy products (milk, cheese, yogurt), fortified plant kinds of milk, leafy green vegetables (kale, broccoli), and almonds.
- **Vitamin D:** Essential for calcium absorption and bone health. Seniors need 800-1,000 IU per day. Natural sources are limited but include fatty fish (salmon, mackerel), egg yolks, and fortified foods. Sunlight exposure also helps the body produce vitamin D.

For Energy:

- **B Vitamins:** Crucial for converting food into energy. This includes B12, B6, thiamine, riboflavin, and niacin. Seniors should ensure adequate intake of these vitamins to support energy levels. Sources include whole grains, meats, fish, eggs, dairy products, and leafy green vegetables. B12 is essential for seniors, with a recommended daily intake of 2.4 µg, since its absorption can decrease with age. Fortified foods or supplements may be necessary.

For Immune Function:

- **Vitamin C:** Vitamin C is known for its role in supporting the immune system. The recommended daily intake is 75 mg for women and 90 mg for men. Sources include citrus fruits, strawberries, bell peppers, and broccoli.
- **Vitamin E:** An antioxidant that helps protect cells from damage and supports immune health. The recommended daily intake is 15 mg. Sources include nuts, seeds, spinach, and broccoli.
- **Zinc:** Important for wound healing and immune function. Seniors need 11 mg (men) and 8 mg (women) daily. Sources include meat, shellfish, legumes, and nuts.
- **Selenium:** Plays a critical role in DNA synthesis and protection from oxidative damage and infection. The recommended intake is 55 µg per day. Sources include Brazil nuts, seafood, and grains.

Hydration: Importance and Guidelines

Hydration remains a cornerstone of health, particularly for seniors, due to age-related changes in the body's water composition and a potentially diminished sense of thirst. Adequate hydration is essential for various bodily functions, including kidney function, regulating body temperature, and maintaining cognitive performance.

- **Understanding Changes in Water Needs:** As we age, the body undergoes several changes that can affect hydration. These include a decrease in total body water, a reduced ability to conserve water, a diminished thirst response, and the use of medications that can impact fluid balance. Consequently, older adults may not feel thirsty until they are already dehydrated. It's essential for seniors and those who care for them to be proactive about maintaining hydration.
- **Guidelines for Adequate Hydration:** Although traditional guidelines suggest eight 8-ounce glasses of water per day, the actual needs

can vary based on factors such as body weight, level of physical activity, climate, and health conditions. A practical approach for seniors is to aim for a minimum of 1.5 to 2 liters of fluids per day, adjusting as needed for individual circumstances. It's crucial to include a variety of fluids and to consider the water content in fruits and vegetables as part of daily intake.

- **Practical Tips for Staying Hydrated:** Establishing regular drinking habits by scheduling times to drink throughout the day ensures a consistent fluid intake, which is crucial before one starts feeling thirsty. Keeping a water bottle or glass within easy reach encourages frequent sipping, thereby facilitating hydration. Additionally, incorporating fluid-rich foods into one's diet, such as cucumbers, strawberries, and melons, can significantly boost overall fluid intake. It's also important to be mindful of diuretics; beverages and foods that can increase fluid loss, such as alcohol and caffeine, should be limited, especially if dehydration is a concern. Moreover, adjusting fluid intake based on activity level and environmental conditions is essential. For instance, in hot weather or during physical activity, seniors should increase their water intake to compensate for the loss through sweat, ensuring adequate hydration.

Understanding and meeting your nutritional needs is a decisive step toward maintaining vitality and health as you age. By focusing on a balanced intake of macronutrients, ensuring you're getting the necessary micronutrients, and staying adequately hydrated, you're setting the stage for active, energized senior years.

As we move forward, remember that nutrition isn't just about what you eat; it's about embracing a lifestyle that supports your body's needs, enabling you to enjoy your senior years to the fullest.

Special Nutritional Considerations for Seniors

As we age, our bodies undergo many changes, impacting everything from how we digest food to how our metabolism processes nutrients. Understanding these changes is crucial for maintaining health and vitality for seniors, especially those leading active lifestyles. This chapter delves into the joint and unique nutritional challenges seniors face, offering insights into how aging affects digestion, metabolism, the management of chronic conditions through diet, decreased appetite, dysphagia, and financial limits. By adapting dietary habits, seniors can enhance their digestive health, adjust to changes in metabolic rate, use nutrition as a tool to manage and mitigate common age-related conditions, stimulate their appetite, find alternatives and modifications to dealing with dysphagia, and maintain a nutritious diet while staying on a budget.

Digestive Changes

Here is a list of changes that affect digestion and nutrient absorption:

- **Decreased Stomach Acid Production:** One of the most significant changes is a reduction in hydrochloric acid production in the stomach. This decrease can lead to challenges in effectively digesting proteins and absorbing vital nutrients such as vitamin B12, iron, and calcium. Since these nutrients are critical in maintaining energy levels, bone health, and overall vitality, their diminished absorption can have notable health implications.
- **Changes in Gastrointestinal Motility:** Aging can also affect food movement through the digestive tract, often slowing it down. This slower transit time can increase the risk of constipation, a common issue among seniors.
- **Alterations in Gut Microbiome:** The composition of the gut microbiome tends to change with age, which can affect digestive health and the immune system. A healthy, diverse gut microbiota is essential for efficient digestion, nutrient absorption, and protection against pathogens.

Strategies to adapt to these changes and support digestive health, seniors can modify their diet in several ways:

- **Increase Fiber Intake:** Consuming a diet high in fiber improves digestion and prevents constipation. Fiber-rich foods include whole grains, vegetables, fruits, and legumes. Aim for 25 to 30 grams of fiber daily, but increase intake gradually to avoid gas and bloating.
- **Stay Hydrated:** Adequate fluid intake is crucial for healthy digestion, helping soften stools and reducing the risk of constipation. As

mentioned in the last chapter, seniors should aim to drink at least eight 8-ounce glasses of water daily, adjusting based on activity level and environmental factors.

- **Incorporate Probiotic and Prebiotic Foods:** Probiotics (found in yogurt, kefir, and fermented foods like sauerkraut and kimchi) can help maintain a healthy gut microbiome. Prebiotic foods like bananas, onions, garlic, and asparagus feed beneficial gut bacteria and support gut health.
- **Mindful of Acidic and Spicy Foods:** Given the decreased stomach acid, some seniors might find that acidic and spicy foods cause discomfort or indigestion. Listening to your body and adjusting your diet can help mitigate these issues.
- **Consider Nutrient-Rich Supplements:** For nutrients that become harder to absorb with age, such as vitamin B12, calcium, and vitamin D, consulting with a healthcare provider about supplementation can ensure adequate intake.

By addressing the digestive changes that come with age through dietary adjustments, seniors can enhance their nutrient absorption, improve digestive health, and enjoy a wide variety of foods as part of a balanced and healthful diet. These strategies not only contribute to better digestive function but also to overall health and well-being.

Metabolic Rate

Overview of Changes in Metabolism with Age: Our basal metabolic rate (BMR) — the number of calories our bodies need to perform essential life-sustaining functions — gradually decreases with age. This decline in BMR is partly due to a loss of muscle mass (sarcopenia) and changes in hormone levels, both common as we age. Additionally, many seniors experience reduced physical activity, contributing to a lower metabolic rate.

Impact on Caloric Needs: A lower BMR and decreased physical activity means that older adults generally need fewer calories to maintain weight than younger people. However, despite needing fewer calories, the need for certain nutrients — such as calcium, vitamin D, and vitamin B12 — may increase, making nutrient-dense foods essential for this age group.

Strategies for adjusting to changes in metabolic rate:

- **Focus on Nutrient Density:** Choose foods with a high nutritional bang for the caloric buck. Examples include fruits, vegetables, lean proteins, whole grains, and low-fat dairy products. These foods can help meet nutrient requirements without excess calorie intake.
- **Maintain Muscle Mass:** Regular physical activity, especially strength training exercises, can help counteract muscle loss and thus help maintain or even slightly increase the metabolic rate.
- **Monitor Portion Sizes:** With a lower caloric requirement, paying attention to portion sizes is essential to avoid unintentional weight gain. Using smaller plates and bowls can help control portions.
- **Stay Hydrated:** Sometimes, thirst is mistaken for hunger. Drinking sufficient water can help manage calorie intake.
- **Eat Regularly:** Skipping meals can further slow down metabolism. Regular, balanced meals help maintain energy levels and metabolic rate.

Managing Chronic Conditions with Diet

Diet plays a pivotal role in managing chronic conditions, particularly those prevalent in senior years, such as heart disease, diabetes, and osteoporosis. By understanding how to adjust your diet, you can significantly mitigate the impact of these conditions, improving your quality of life and overall health.

Heart Disease

Foods to Embrace:

- **Omega-3 Fatty Acids:** Foods rich in omega-3s, such as salmon, mackerel, flaxseeds, and walnuts, can help reduce heart disease risk factors by lowering triglyceride levels and enhancing heart health.
- **Fruits and Vegetables:** A diet high in fruits and vegetables is linked to lower heart disease risk. They're rich in vitamins, minerals, fiber, and antioxidants.
- **Whole Grains:** Foods like whole wheat, brown rice, oats, and barley can improve cholesterol levels and support heart health.

Foods to Avoid:

- **Saturated and Trans Fats:** Limit red meats, butter, cheese, and processed foods to reduce bad cholesterol levels.
- **Excessive Salt:** High sodium intake can increase blood pressure. Aim for less than 2,300 mg daily, or even lower if possible.

Diabetes

Foods to Embrace:

- **Low-Glycemic Index Foods:** Foods that have a minimal impact on blood glucose levels, such as leafy greens, whole grains, and legumes, are beneficial for managing diabetes.
- **Lean Proteins:** Incorporate lean proteins such as chicken, fish, tofu, and beans to help manage hunger and blood sugar levels.
- **Healthy Fats:** Avocados, nuts, and seeds contain fats that can help slow sugar absorption into the bloodstream.

Foods to Avoid:

- **Refined Sugars and Carbohydrates:** Foods high in refined sugars and white flour can cause rapid spikes in blood glucose levels. Avoid sugary drinks, pastries, and white bread.
- **Processed Snacks:** Many processed foods are high in unhealthy fats, sugars, and salt, which can disrupt blood sugar management.

Osteoporosis

Foods to Embrace:

- **Calcium-Rich Foods:** Dairy products, fortified plant kinds of milk, leafy greens, and almonds are excellent sources of calcium, essential for bone health.
- **Vitamin D:** It helps the body absorb calcium. Sources include fatty fish, egg yolks, fortified foods, and sensible sun exposure.

Foods to Avoid:

- **Excessive Sodium:** High sodium intake can cause calcium loss, negatively affecting bone density. Limit processed and canned foods.
- **High-Caffeine Beverages:** While moderate caffeine consumption is generally safe, excessive intake can interfere with calcium absorption.

Decreased Appetite

A decrease in appetite can have various causes, including changes in taste and smell, side effects of medications, psychological factors such as depression or loneliness, and decreased physical activity. Addressing decreased appetite is crucial for preventing malnutrition and maintaining overall health.

Strategies to manage decreased appetite:

- **Enhance Flavor Without Adding Salt or Sugar:** As the sense of taste may diminish with age, enhancing the flavor of foods can make eating more appealing. Use a variety of herbs, spices, and healthy fats like olive oil to add richness and depth to dishes. Lemon juice, vinegar, and aromatic herbs can also make meals more enticing without resorting to excessive salt or sugar.
- **Create Enjoyable Eating Environments:** Eating in a pleasant, social setting can stimulate appetite. Sharing meals with friends or family whenever possible or participating in community dining events can make mealtime more of an occasion and less of a chore.
- **Prioritize Nutrient-Dense Foods:** Focusing on foods that pack a high nutritional punch is necessary when appetite is limited. Incorporate a variety of colorful fruits and vegetables, whole grains, lean proteins, and healthy fats into your diet. Smoothies and soups

can be beneficial for incorporating multiple nutrient sources in an easy-to-consume format.

- **Listen to Your Body:** Eat when you're most hungry, even if it's not a traditional mealtime. Make breakfast your largest meal if you feel more hungry in the morning. Conversely, plan a substantial, nutritious dinner if evenings find you hungrier.
- **Small, Frequent Meals:** Large meals can be overwhelming when your appetite is small. Instead, aim for smaller portions spread out over the day. This not only can help with managing appetite but also assists in maintaining steady energy levels and nutrient intake.
- **Stay Hydrated with Nutritious Liquids:** Sometimes, solid foods may seem unappealing. Nutritious liquids such as vegetable juices, milk, or smoothies enriched with protein powder can provide essential nutrients and help maintain hydration.
- **Consult Healthcare Providers:** If decreased appetite is a persistent issue, it could indicate an underlying health condition. Consulting a healthcare provider can help identify specific causes and determine the best action to address them. They can also recommend appetite stimulants or supplements if needed.

Dysphagia

Dysphagia, or difficulty chewing or swallowing, can significantly affect seniors' ability to consume various foods, potentially leading to nutritional deficiencies. This condition might stem from dental issues, muscular or neurological disorders, or changes in the mouth and throat's structure. Ensuring adequate nutrition despite these challenges is crucial for maintaining health and quality of life.

Strategies to manage difficulty chewing or swallowing:

- **Opt for Soft Foods and Liquids:** Incorporate soft foods that require minimal chewing, such as mashed potatoes, scrambled eggs, well-cooked pasta, oatmeal, and ripe bananas. Soups and smoothies can also provide necessary nutrients in an easily consumable form.
- **Modify Food Textures:** If certain foods are essential for nutrition but challenging to chew or swallow, consider modifying their texture. Vegetables can be steamed and pureed, meats can be ground or finely chopped and mixed into soups or casseroles, and fruits can be blended into smoothies or made into sauces.
- **Stay Hydrated:** Proper hydration is essential, especially for those with swallowing difficulties, to help facilitate the swallowing process. Thicker liquids such as smoothies, milkshakes, or even specialized thickened beverages can be easier to swallow for some individuals.
- **Use Specialized Eating Utensils:** Utensils designed for individuals with swallowing difficulties can make a significant difference. Tools like sippy cups, straws, or utensils with easy-grip handles can aid in self-feeding and independence.
- **Practice Safe Swallowing Techniques:** Certain techniques can make swallowing safer and easier. These include taking smaller bites, eating slowly, and sitting upright during and after meals. A speech-language pathologist can provide specific exercises and strategies tailored to individual needs.
- **Regular Dental Care:** Regular checkups and care are essential for those whose chewing difficulties are related to dental issues. Dentures should be well-fitted and adjusted as necessary to aid in chewing.
- **Consult Healthcare Professionals:** A multidisciplinary approach involving dietitians, speech-language pathologists, and healthcare providers is often necessary to address the underlying causes of chewing or swallowing difficulties. These professionals can also

recommend appropriate dietary modifications, supplements, or therapeutic interventions to ensure adequate nutrition.

Financial Constraints

Financial constraints can significantly impact the ability to maintain a nutritious diet, especially for seniors living on fixed incomes. Limited budgets may restrict access to various healthy foods, mainly fresh fruits, vegetables, and lean proteins, which are often more expensive than processed options. Addressing the challenge of eating well within financial limitations is crucial for ensuring seniors can continue supporting their health and well-being without financial strain.

Strategies to manage nutrition on a budget:

- **Plan Meals in Advance:** Planning meals for the week can help avoid impulse buys and ensure that purchases are limited to what's necessary, reducing waste and saving money. Look for sales and discounts in local store flyers or apps and plan meals around what's on offer.
- **Buy in Bulk:** Purchasing non-perishable items like whole grains, legumes, and canned goods in bulk can save money in the long run. These items are nutritious, have a long shelf life, and can serve as the foundation for multiple meals.
- **Choose Frozen or Canned Produce:** Frozen and canned fruits and vegetables can be more affordable than fresh produce and are just as nutritious. Opt for those without added sugars or sodium. They can be a great way to ensure you're getting enough fruits and vegetables in your diet.
- **Use Coupons and Loyalty Programs:** Many grocery stores offer loyalty programs that provide discounts to members. Combining

coupons with these discounts can lead to significant savings on grocery bills.

- **Cook at Home:** Preparing meals at home is generally more cost-effective than eating out. Cooking in batches can save time and ensure that healthy options are always available.
- **Embrace Plant-Based Proteins:** Plant-based proteins such as beans, lentils, and chickpeas are often less expensive than animal proteins and can provide similar nutritional benefits. Incorporating these into meals several times a week can reduce grocery bills while supporting a balanced diet.
- **Community Resources:** Look into community resources like senior meal programs, food banks, or subsidized grocery programs designed to help those on fixed incomes access nutritious foods. Local community gardens can also produce fresh produce during the growing season.
- **Grow Your Own:** Growing your fruits, vegetables, and herbs can be a cost-effective way to supplement your diet with fresh produce. Even those with limited space can grow herbs on a windowsill or tomatoes in a patio container.

4

Meal Planning and Preparation

Navigating the world of nutrition as an active senior can be a simple puzzle. This chapter simplifies the process, offering a roadmap to crafting meal plans that fulfill your nutritional needs, suggesting nutritious snacks for sustained energy, sharing easy recipes for wholesome meals, and demonstrating how to enrich your diet with nutrient-dense foods. Integrating these practices into your daily routine allows you to enjoy delicious, healthy meals supporting an active, vibrant lifestyle.

Planning Balanced Meals

Creating balanced meals is an excellent way for seniors to maintain an active lifestyle. A well-planned meal nourishes your body and supports your physical and mental well-being. Here, we delve into how to construct meal plans that seamlessly incorporate all the necessary nutrients, ensuring you're fueled for the day ahead.

Sample Meal Plan 1

Breakfast: Avocado toast on one slice of whole-grain bread, topped with half a sliced avocado, a side of 1/2 cup cottage cheese, and a medium-sized sliced peach. This meal provides healthy fats, protein, fiber, and vitamins.

Lunch: Turkey and hummus wrap using one whole-grain tortilla, 3 ounces of sliced turkey breast, two tablespoons of hummus, mixed greens, shredded carrots, and slices of red bell pepper. Serve with one medium apple on the side for added fiber and vitamins.

Dinner: Baked lemon-garlic chicken breast (about 4 ounces), served with 1/2 cup cooked quinoa and a cup of steamed green beans topped with a tablespoon of sliced almonds, offering a balanced mix of protein, carbs, and healthy fats.

Sample Meal Plan 2

Breakfast: 1 cup of Greek yogurt mixed with a tablespoon of ground flaxseed, a teaspoon of honey, and a cup of mixed fresh berries (strawberries, blueberries, raspberries), providing protein, omega-3s, and antioxidants.

Lunch: Lentil soup with 1 cup of lentils and a cup of mixed vegetables (spinach, carrots, tomatoes) served with a slice of whole-grain bread, rich in protein, fiber, and essential nutrients.

Dinner: Stir-fried tofu (about 3.5 ounces) with a cup each of broccoli, bell peppers, and snap peas served over 1/2 cup of cooked brown rice. This meal is high in plant-based protein and offers many vitamins.

Sample Meal Plan 3

Breakfast: Scrambled eggs (made with two eggs) with spinach and tomatoes, served with one whole-grain English muffin. This meal combines high-quality protein with fiber and essential vitamins.

Lunch: Quinoa salad with 1/2 cup cooked quinoa, 1/4 cup chickpeas, diced cucumber, cherry tomatoes, and feta cheese, dressed with olive oil and lemon juice. It's a fiber-rich meal with healthy fats and protein.

Dinner: Grilled salmon (about 4 ounces) served with a side salad (mixed greens, a handful of walnuts, slices of avocado, and vinaigrette) and 1/2 cup roasted sweet potatoes. This meal offers omega-3 fatty acids, healthy fats, and complex carbs.

Pro Tips

- **Portion Control:** Use your hand as a guide for portion sizes: a fist for vegetables, a palm-sized portion for proteins, a cupped hand for carbs, and a thumb for fats.
- **Stay Flexible:** Be willing to swap ingredients based on availability and personal preference. Nutrition is not one-size-fits-all.
- **Mindful Eating:** Pay attention to hunger and fullness cues to avoid overeating. Enjoy your food and the experience of eating.
- **Hydration:** Remember to drink water throughout the day. Aim for about 8 glasses, but adjust according to your activity level and environment.

Healthy Snacking

For active seniors, healthy snacking is crucial for maintaining energy levels, supporting overall health, and filling nutritional gaps between meals. Snacks can provide an excellent opportunity to incorporate more vitamins, minerals, and other essential nutrients into your diet. Here are several nutritious snack ideas designed to support an active lifestyle, complete with suggested portion sizes to help manage energy and maintain a balanced diet.

Snack Ideas

- **Fruit and Nut Butter:** Pair a medium apple or banana with 1 tablespoon of almond or peanut butter. This combination offers a good mix of carbohydrates for energy, protein, and healthy fats for satiety and muscle repair.
- **Greek Yogurt and Berries:** Enjoy 3/4 cup of plain Greek yogurt topped with 1/2 cup of mixed berries. Greek yogurt is high in protein, and berries provide antioxidants and a sweet flavor with minimal added sugars.
- **Vegetable Sticks and Hummus:** Cut up a cup of mixed vegetables, such as carrots, cucumbers, and bell peppers, and dip in 2 tablespoons of hummus. This snack is rich in fiber and vitamins from the vegetables and provides protein and healthy fats from the hummus.
- **Whole Grain Crackers and Cheese:** Have 3-4 whole grain crackers with 1 ounce of cheese. This pairing offers a satisfying crunch with the crackers and protein and calcium from the cheese.
- **Nuts and Dried Fruit:** For a quick, energy-boosting snack, mix a small handful (about 1 ounce or 1/4 cup) of nuts, such as almonds or walnuts, with a tablespoon of dried fruit. Nuts provide healthy fats, protein, and fiber, while dried fruit offers natural sweetness and a quick energy source.
- **Roasted Chickpeas:** 1/4 cup of roasted chickpeas can be a crunchy, protein-rich snack. They're also high in fiber, satisfying and great for digestive health.

- **Cottage Cheese and Pineapple:** Combine 1/2 cup of cottage cheese with 1/2 cup of chopped pineapple. This snack offers protein from the cottage cheese and vitamins from the pineapple.
- **Hard-Boiled Eggs:** 1-2 hard-boiled eggs make a protein-packed snack that's easy to prepare in advance. Eggs are also a good source of vitamin D and B vitamins.

Snacking Tips

- **Portion Control:** Stick to the suggested portion sizes to manage calorie intake and prevent overeating.
- **Prepare in Advance:** Pre-portion snacks or prepare them ahead of time to grab-and-go, making it easier to choose healthy options.
- **Listen to Your Body:** Snack when you're genuinely hungry rather than out of boredom or habit, and choose snacks that satisfy your cravings while providing nutritional value.
- **Stay Hydrated:** Sometimes, thirst is mistaken for hunger. Drink a glass of water before snacking to ensure you're starving.

Cooking and Preparation Tips

Eating healthily doesn't have to involve complex recipes or long hours in the kitchen. With simple cooking techniques and ingredient choices, you can prepare nutritious, delicious meals that support an active senior lifestyle. Below are easy-to-follow recipes and tips to enhance the nutrient density of your meals, along with guidance on portion sizes.

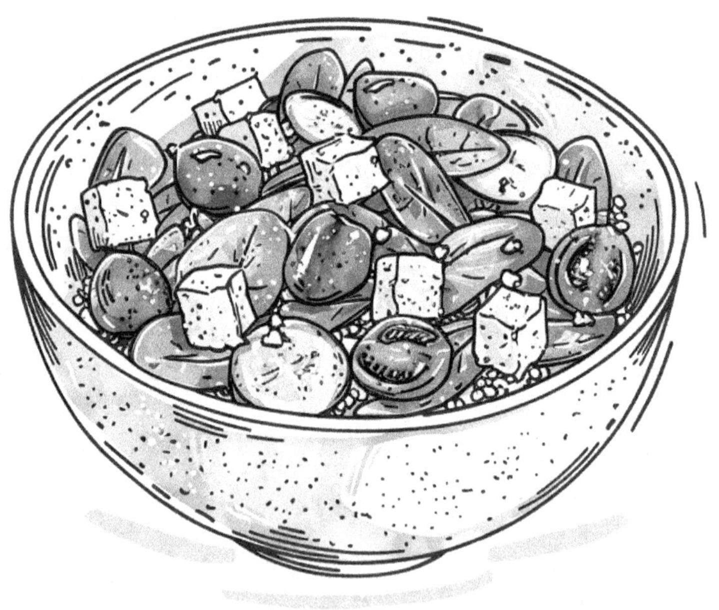

Quinoa Vegetable Salad

Ingredients:

- 1 cup cooked quinoa
- 1 cup chopped spinach
- 1/2 cup cherry tomatoes (halved)

- 1/4 cup diced cucumber
- 1/4 cup feta cheese
- 2 tablespoons olive oil
- 1 tablespoon lemon juice, salt, and pepper to taste.

Instructions:

1. In a large bowl, combine the cooked quinoa, chopped spinach, cherry tomatoes, and cucumber.
2. Drizzle with olive oil and lemon juice. Toss to combine.
3. Sprinkle feta cheese on top and season with salt and pepper to taste.
4. Serve chilled or at room temperature.

Portion Size: Serves 2. For a balanced meal rich in fiber, protein, and healthy fats, serve half the prepared salad per person.

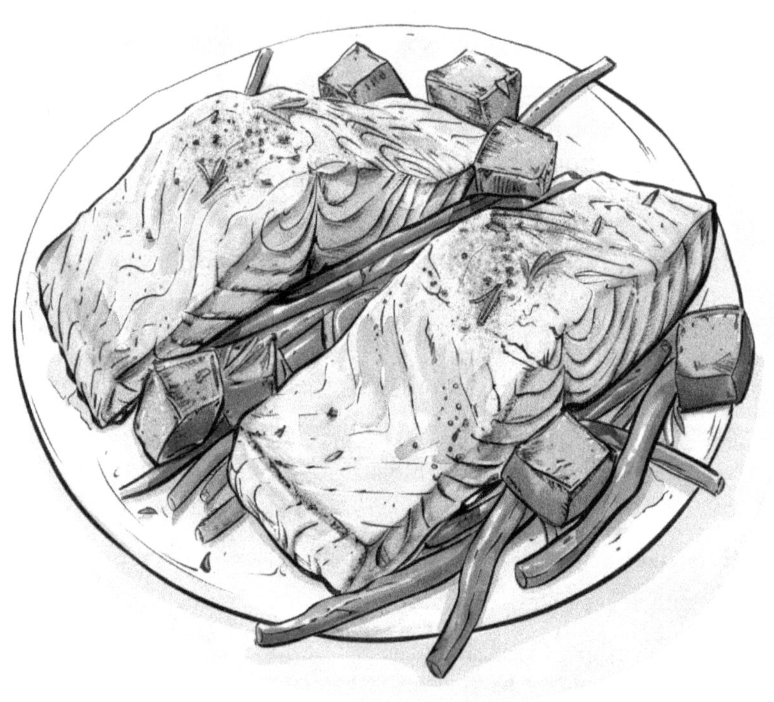

Baked Salmon with Sweet Potato and Green Beans

Ingredients:

- 2 salmon filets (about 4 oz each)
- 1 large sweet potato (cubed)
- 1 cup green beans (trimmed)
- 2 tablespoons olive oil
- 1 teaspoon paprika, salt, and pepper to taste.

Instructions:

1. Preheat your oven to 400°F (200°C). Line a baking sheet with parchment paper.
2. Toss the sweet potato cubes with half the olive oil, paprika, salt, and pepper. Spread them out on one side of the baking sheet.
3. Place the salmon filets on the other side of the sheet. Drizzle with the remaining olive oil and season with salt and pepper.
4. Scatter the green beans around the salmon and sweet potatoes.
5. Bake for 20-25 minutes, until the salmon is cooked through and the vegetables are tender.

Portion Size: Serves 2. This meal provides balanced protein, complex carbs, and vegetables.

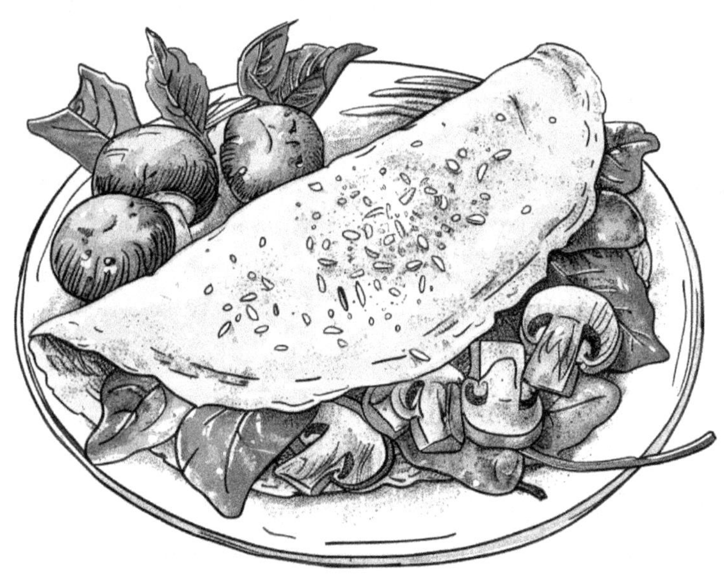

Spinach and Mushroom Omelet

Ingredients:

- 2 eggs
- 1 cup fresh spinach
- 1/2 cup sliced mushrooms
- 1 tablespoon grated cheese (optional)
- Salt and pepper to taste
- 1 teaspoon olive oil

Instructions:

1. Heat olive oil in a skillet over medium heat. Sauté mushrooms until soft.
2. Add spinach and cook until wilted. Remove vegetables from the skillet.
3. Beat eggs with salt and pepper, then pour into the skillet. Cook until the edges start to set.
4. Place the sautéed vegetables on one half of the omelet. Sprinkle with cheese if using.
5. Fold the omelet over the vegetables, cook for another minute, then serve.

Portion Size: Serves 1. Provides a good balance of protein, healthy fats, and vegetables.

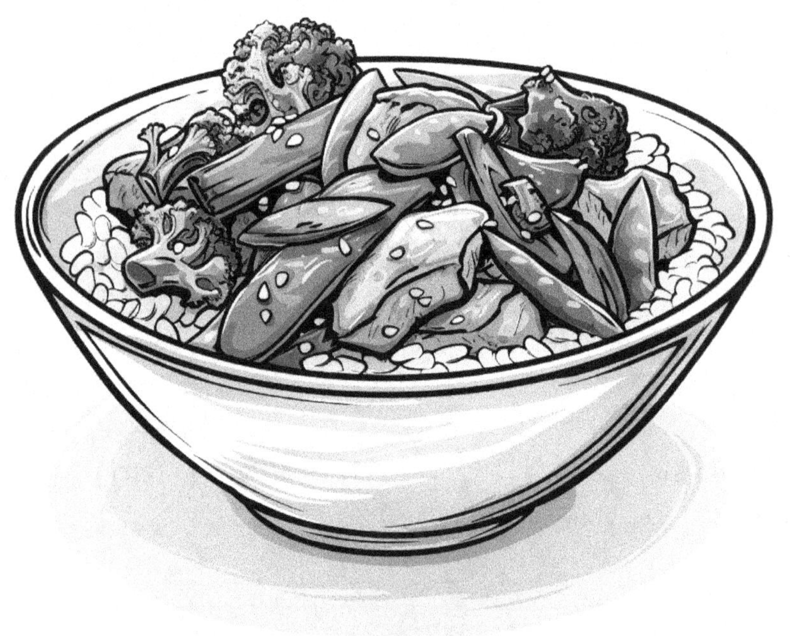

Chicken and Veggie Stir-fry

Ingredients:

- 4 oz chicken breast, thinly sliced
- 1 cup broccoli florets
- 1/2 cup sliced bell pepper
- 1/2 cup snap peas
- 2 tablespoons low-sodium soy sauce
- 1 teaspoon sesame oil
- 1 garlic clove, minced
- 1/2 cup cooked brown rice

Instructions:

1. Heat sesame oil in a pan over medium-high heat. Add garlic and sauté for 30 seconds.
2. Add chicken slices and cook until no longer pink.
3. Add vegetables and soy sauce. Stir-fry until vegetables are tender but crisp.
4. Serve over cooked brown rice.

Portion Size: Serves 1. Offers a complete meal with lean protein, whole grains, and various vegetables.

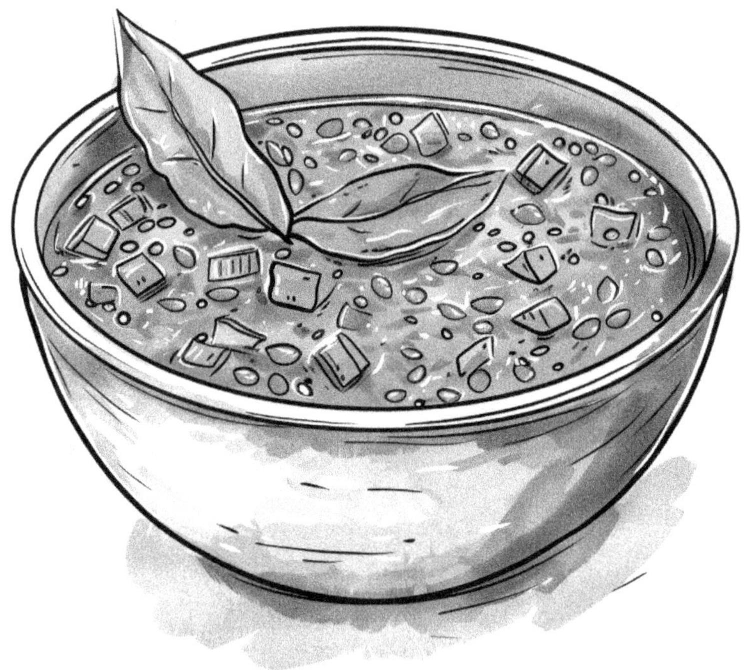

Lentil Soup

Ingredients:

- 1/2 cup dried lentils
- 2 cups vegetable broth
- 1/2 cup diced carrots
- 1/2 cup diced celery
- 1/2 cup diced tomatoes
- 1 teaspoon olive oil
- Salt and pepper to taste
- 1 bay leaf (optional)

Instructions:

1. Heat olive oil in a pot over medium heat. Add carrots and celery, sautéing until softened.
2. Add lentils, tomatoes, vegetable broth, bay leaf, salt, and pepper.
3. Bring to a boil, then reduce heat and simmer until lentils are tender about 20-25 minutes.
4. Remove bay leaf and serve.

Portion Size: Serves 2. A hearty and nutritious soup rich in protein, fiber, and vitamins.

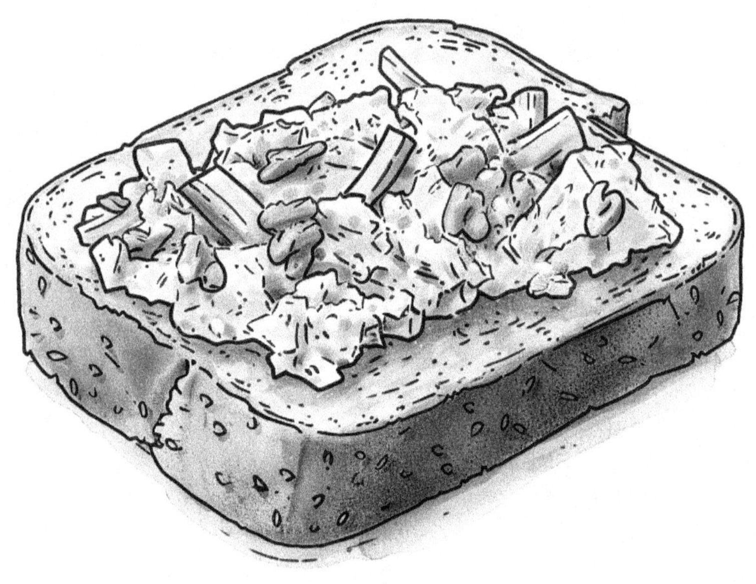

Tuna Salad on Whole Grain Bread

Ingredients:

- 4 oz canned tuna in water, drained
- 2 tablespoons Greek yogurt
- 1/4 cup diced celery
- 1 tablespoon chopped walnuts
- Salt and pepper to taste
- 2 slices whole-grain bread

Instructions:

1. In a bowl, mix tuna, Greek yogurt, celery, walnuts, salt, and pepper.
2. Spread the mixture on one slice of bread, top with the other slice, and serve.

Portion Size: Serves 1. A balanced sandwich with lean protein, healthy fats, and whole grains.

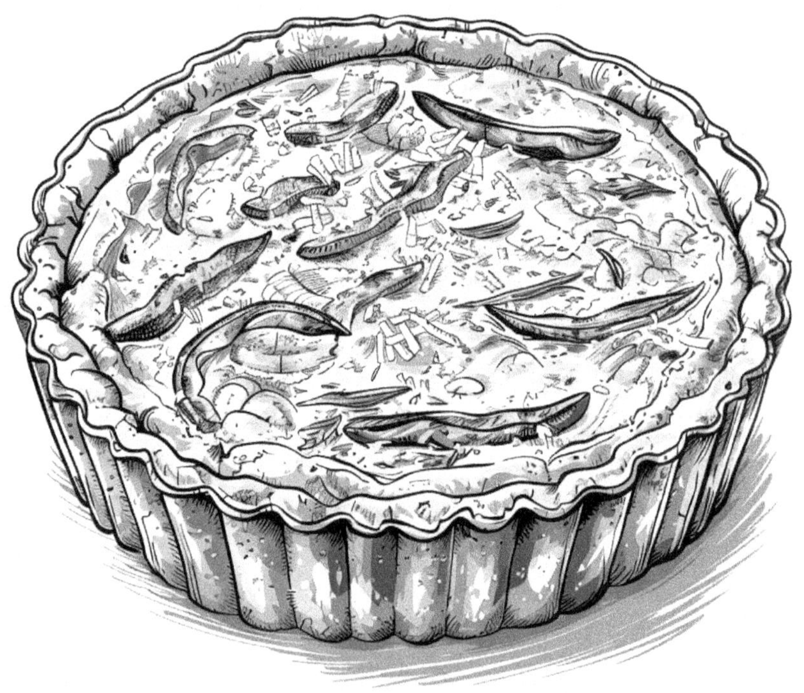

Roasted Vegetable Quiche

Ingredients:

- 1 cup mixed vegetables (zucchini, bell peppers, onions), chopped
- 4 eggs
- 1/4 cup milk
- 1/2 cup shredded cheese (optional)
- Salt and pepper to taste
- 1 pre-made whole-grain pie crust (optional)

Instructions:

1. Preheat the oven to 375°F (190°C). Roast chopped vegetables on a baking sheet until tender, about 20 minutes.
2. Whisk together eggs, milk, salt, and pepper.
3. Spread roasted vegetables evenly over the pie crust (if using), pour the egg mixture on top, and sprinkle with cheese.
4. Bake for 25-30 minutes or until the quiche is set and lightly browned.

Portion Size: Serves 4. A nutritious quiche offering a good balance of vegetables, protein, and whole grains (if using a crust).

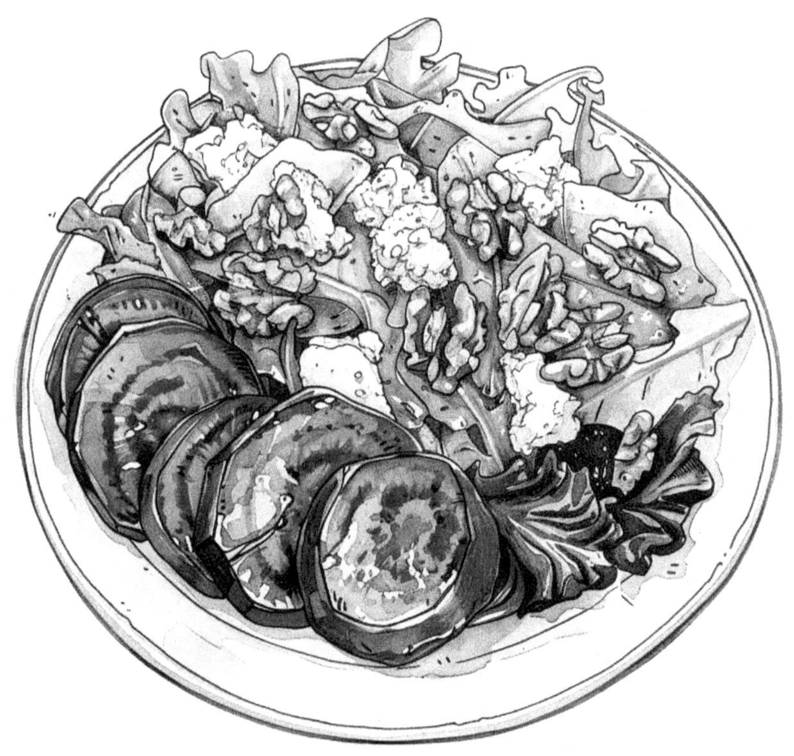

Beet and Goat Cheese Salad

Ingredients:

- 2 medium beets, roasted and sliced
- 2 cups mixed greens
- 1/4 cup crumbled goat cheese
- 2 tablespoons chopped walnuts
- 2 tablespoons balsamic vinaigrette

Instructions:

1. Arrange mixed greens on a plate. Top with sliced beets, goat cheese, and walnuts.
2. Drizzle with balsamic vinaigrette before serving.

Portion Size: Serves 2. This salad is an excellent source of vitamins, minerals, and healthy fats.

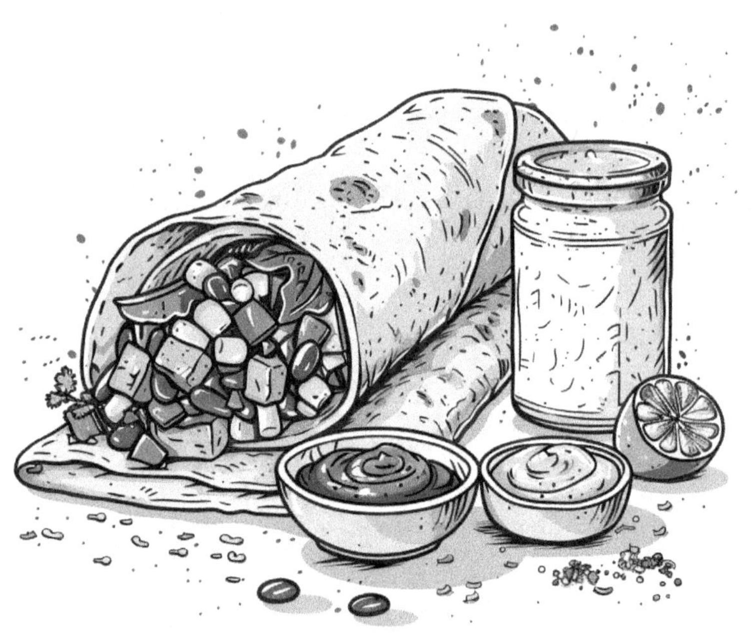

Sweet Potato and Black Bean Burritos

Ingredients:

- 1 medium sweet potato, peeled and diced
- 1/2 cup black beans, rinsed and drained
- 1/4 cup corn (frozen or fresh)
- 1/2 teaspoon cumin
- Salt and pepper to taste
- 2 whole wheat tortillas
- 1/4 cup shredded cheese (optional)
- 2 tablespoons Greek yogurt (for serving)

- 1/4 cup salsa (for serving)

Instructions:

1. Boil or steam the sweet potato cubes until tender, about 15 minutes.
2. In a bowl, mix the cooked sweet potato, black beans, corn, cumin, salt, and pepper.
3. Divide the mixture evenly between the two tortillas. Top with shredded cheese if using.
4. Roll up the tortillas, folding in the sides to enclose the filling.
5. Heat a skillet over medium heat. Place the burritos seam-side down and cook until golden brown on both sides.
6. Serve with Greek yogurt and salsa on the side.

Portion Size: Serves 2. Each burrito provides a balanced mix of complex carbs, protein, and healthy fats, making it a filling and nutritious meal option.

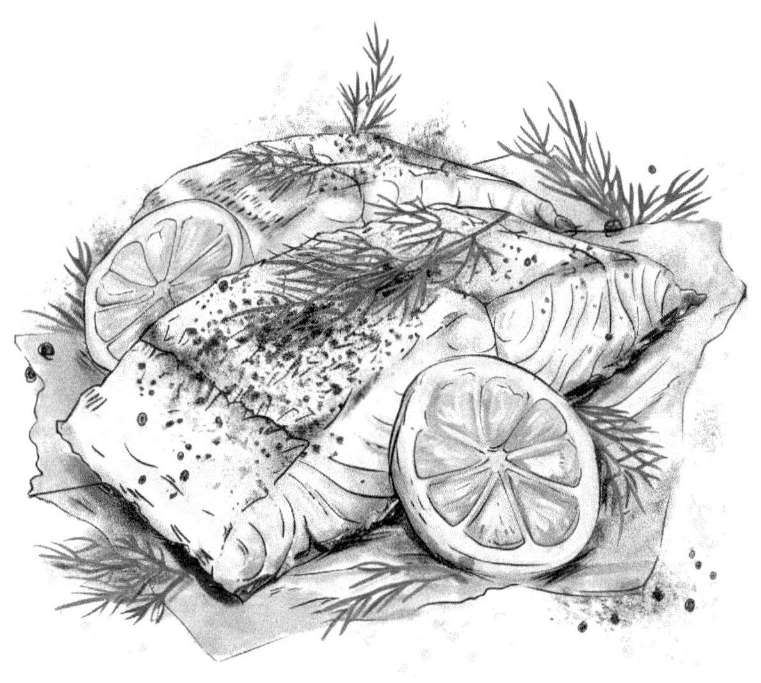

Baked Cod with Lemon and Dill

Ingredients:

- 2 cod filets (about 4 oz each)
- 1 tablespoon olive oil
- 1 lemon, sliced
- 1 teaspoon dried dill or 1 tablespoon fresh dill
- Salt and pepper to taste

Instructions:

1. Preheat the oven to 400°F (200°C). Line a baking sheet with parchment paper.
2. Place the cod filets on the baking sheet. Drizzle with olive oil and season with salt, pepper, and dill.
3. Top each filet with a few lemon slices.
4. Bake for 12-15 minutes or until the fish flakes easily with a fork.
5. Serve immediately, garnished with additional lemon slices if desired.

Portion Size: Serves 2. This dish is light yet satisfying, offering a good source of lean protein and healthy fats, along with the refreshing flavors of lemon and dill.

Making Meals More Nutrient-Dense

- **Add Veggies:** Bulk up meals with vegetables. Add spinach to smoothies, mix grated carrots or zucchini into pasta sauces, or top pizzas with arugula after baking.
- **Choose Whole Grains:** Swap refined grains for whole grains. For example, use brown rice instead of white, whole-grain pasta, and bread to increase fiber and nutrients.
- **Protein Boost:** Incorporate lean protein into each meal. Add chickpeas to salads, snack on Greek yogurt, or have a piece of chicken or fish as part of your main meal.
- **Healthy Fats:** Include sources of healthy fats for their heart-health benefits. Sprinkle nuts or seeds on salads, use avocado in sandwiches, and cook with olive oil.
- **Herbs and Spices:** Herbs and spices enhance flavor and nutrient content without adding extra calories. Turmeric, ginger, garlic, and

cinnamon all add flavor and offer health benefits.

Focusing on these simple recipes and tips for making meals more nutrient-dense can help you enjoy delicious, healthy meals that support your active lifestyle. The key to a balanced diet is variety, so feel free to adjust recipes and ingredients according to your preferences and nutritional needs.

5

Supplements for Active Seniors

As we progress through life stages, our nutritional needs evolve, and maintaining an optimal nutrient intake becomes increasingly crucial for sustaining an active and healthy lifestyle. Despite our best efforts to consume a balanced and nutrient-dense diet, there may still be gaps that could affect our overall health and vitality. Supplements can be pivotal in bridging these nutritional gaps, but it's essential to approach supplementation with knowledge and caution. This chapter explores the necessity of supplements for active seniors, highlights various types of crucial supplements, and addresses the risks and recommendations associated with their use.

When Supplements Are Necessary

For active seniors, maintaining optimal nutrition is not just about eating a balanced diet—it's about ensuring the body receives all the nutrients it needs to function at its best. Despite efforts to consume a varied and nutrient-dense diet, certain conditions and age-related changes can create gaps in nutrition that might necessitate supplementation. Identifying and addressing these gaps is crucial for sustaining health, vitality, and an active lifestyle as we age.

Identifying Nutritional Gaps:

- **Dietary Restrictions:** Seniors who adhere to specific dietary restrictions, such as vegetarian or vegan diets, may find it challenging to obtain adequate amounts of certain nutrients, including vitamin B12, iron, and omega-3 fatty acids, predominantly found in animal products.
- **Reduced Nutrient Absorption:** Age-related changes in the gastrointestinal system can lead to decreased absorption of critical nutrients. For example, the body's ability to absorb vitamin B12 declines with age, impacting energy levels and cognitive function.
- **Increased Nutritional Needs:** Certain health conditions common in older adults, such as osteoporosis, require an increased intake of specific nutrients like calcium and vitamin D to maintain bone density. Similarly, conditions like age-related macular degeneration may benefit from higher levels of antioxidants, such as lutein and zeaxanthin.

Evaluating the Need for Supplements:

- **Regular Nutritional Assessments:** Routine dietary assessments can help identify potential nutrient deficiencies. These assessments should consider dietary intake, lifestyle factors, and health conditions or medications affecting nutrient absorption or requirements.
- **Blood Tests:** Blood tests can provide a clear picture of nutrient levels in the body, pinpointing specific deficiencies. Standard tests include levels of vitamin D, vitamin B12, iron, and calcium.
- **Symptoms of Deficiency:** Awareness of the signs and symptoms of nutrient deficiencies is crucial. For instance, fatigue and

weakness could indicate an iron deficiency, while brittle bones and frequent fractures may suggest inadequate calcium and vitamin D intake.

Valuable Insights:

- **Supplementation as a Tool, Not a Replacement:** Supplements should complement a healthy diet, not replace it. They fill specific nutritional gaps rather than provide the primary source of nutrients.
- **Personalized Approach:** Because nutritional needs vary widely among individuals, supplement regimens should be tailored to the individual's specific dietary habits, health status, and nutritional requirements.

In summary, supplements can play a vital role in the nutritional strategy of active seniors, especially when dietary restrictions, decreased nutrient absorption, and increased nutritional needs create gaps that are difficult to fill through diet alone. Recognizing when these gaps exist and taking steps to address them with a thoughtful, evidence-based supplementation approach can help ensure seniors maintain the nutrient levels necessary for optimal health and activity.

Types of Supplements

Supplements can serve as crucial allies in an active senior's quest for optimal health, particularly when addressing specific nutritional gaps. Among the array of supplements available, multivitamins, calcium, vitamin D, omega-3 fatty acids, and protein supplements stand out for their broad health benefits and importance in senior nutrition. A closer look at each of these supplement types reveals their unique roles and the insights they offer into maintaining wellness in later years.

Multivitamins

- **Overview:** Multivitamins are comprehensive supplements designed to provide a wide range of essential vitamins and minerals in one product. They serve as a nutritional safety net, helping to ensure that daily nutrient requirements are met, significantly when dietary intake may fall short.
- **Benefits for Seniors:** Multivitamins can be particularly beneficial in filling nutritional gaps due to dietary limitations or increased needs. They can support overall health, bolster the immune system, and contribute to better cognitive function.
- **Considerations:** While multivitamins complement a balanced diet, they cannot replicate whole foods' complex mix of nutrients and phytochemicals. It is crucial to choose a multivitamin tailored to the nutritional needs of seniors, with appropriate levels of vitamin D, vitamin B12, and calcium.

Calcium

- **Overview:** Calcium is vital for maintaining strong bones and teeth, supporting muscle function, and ensuring proper nerve transmission. As bone density naturally decreases with age, calcium's role becomes even more critical.
- **Benefits for Seniors:** Adequate calcium intake can help mitigate the risk of osteoporosis, a condition prevalent among older adults that leads to increased fragility and fracture risk.
- **Considerations:** While dairy products are a primary calcium source, supplements can help seniors who are lactose intolerant or have dietary preferences that limit calcium intake. Not exceeding

recommended doses is essential, as too much calcium can lead to kidney stones and impaired absorption of other minerals.

Vitamin D

- **Overview:** Vitamin D is pivotal in calcium absorption, bone health, immune function, and inflammation reduction. The body's ability to synthesize vitamin D from sunlight decreases with age, making supplementation more relevant for seniors.
- **Benefits for Seniors:** Supplementing with vitamin D can support bone health, reduce the risk of falls and fractures, and may have protective effects against certain cancers and heart disease.
- **Considerations:** Vitamin D supplementation is essential in regions with limited sunlight exposure and for individuals with limited outdoor activities. Blood tests can help determine the appropriate supplementation level to correct or prevent deficiency.

Omega-3 Fatty Acids

- **Overview:** Omega-3 fatty acids are essential fats the body cannot produce alone. They are crucial for heart health, brain function, and reducing inflammation.
- **Benefits for Seniors:** Omega-3 supplements, such as fish oil, can support cardiovascular health, aid in cognitive function, and may help reduce symptoms of rheumatoid arthritis.
- **Considerations:** Omega-3s are most commonly found in fatty fish, but supplements can provide a convenient alternative for those who don't consume fish. Choosing high-quality, mercury-free omega-3 supplements is essential to ensure safety and efficacy.

Protein Supplements

- **Overview:** Protein supplements come in various forms, including powders, shakes, and bars, and are derived from different sources such as whey, casein, soy, and peas. Protein is crucial for muscle repair, bone health, and maintaining lean muscle mass, which tends to decrease with age.
- **Benefits for Seniors:** Protein supplements can be valuable for active seniors in supporting muscle recovery after exercise, maintaining muscle strength, and ensuring adequate daily protein intake when dietary sources may be insufficient. Adequate protein is also essential for injury recovery and immune system function.
- **Considerations:** While whole food protein sources are preferred for their additional nutritional benefits, protein supplements can offer a convenient and efficient way to meet increased protein needs, particularly post-exercise or for seniors with higher protein requirements due to health conditions. Choosing high-quality protein supplements without excessive added sugars or artificial ingredients is essential. The type of protein supplement (e.g., whey for quick absorption post-workout, casein for slow release before bed) should match the individual's health goals and dietary restrictions.

Risks and Recommendations

While dietary supplements offer numerous benefits, especially for active seniors seeking to fill nutritional gaps or support overall health, they are not without risks. Understanding how to navigate these risks and make informed choices is crucial. This section provides insights into the potential risks associated with supplement use, offers recommendations for selecting the right supplements, and discusses the importance of consulting healthcare providers.

Understanding the Risks

Interactions with Medications: Some supplements can interact with prescription medications, either reducing their effectiveness or enhancing their effects, which can lead to adverse outcomes. For example, supplements like vitamin K can affect blood thinners, while supplements such as St. John's Wort can interfere with antidepressants.

Overconsumption: Consuming higher doses of vitamins and minerals than the body needs can lead to toxicity and health issues. Fat-soluble vitamins (A, D, E, and K) are particularly concerning because they are stored in the body's fat tissues and can accumulate to toxic levels over time.

Quality and Purity Concerns: The dietary supplement industry is vast and varied, with significant differences in the quality and purity of products. Some supplements may not contain the advertised amount of active ingredients, and others may be contaminated with harmful substances.

Recommendations for Choosing the Right Supplements

Research and Education: Before adding any supplement to your regimen, research its benefits, potential side effects, and interactions with the medications you're taking. Look for scientific studies and reputable sources of information to guide your decisions.

Quality Assurance: Opt for supplements verified by third-party organizations such as USP (United States Pharmacopeia) or NSF International, which test supplements for quality and purity.

Personalized Approach: When choosing supplements, consider your dietary intake, lifestyle, and specific health needs. What works for one person may not be appropriate for another. Tailoring your supplement choices to your individual needs can maximize benefits and minimize risks.

The Importance of Consulting Healthcare Providers for Supplements

Expert Guidance: Healthcare providers can offer personalized advice based on a comprehensive understanding of your health status, dietary habits, and medication regimen. They can identify potential nutrient deficiencies, recommend appropriate supplements, and monitor their effectiveness and safety.

Medication Interactions: A healthcare provider can help you understand possible interactions between supplements and medications, adjusting dosages or recommending alternative treatments as necessary.

Ongoing Evaluation: Nutritional needs and health conditions can change over time. Regular consultations with healthcare providers ensure your supplement regimen aligns with your current health needs and goals.

Incorporating supplements into your health regimen as an active senior can significantly contribute to your nutritional well-being and overall health. However, navigating the risks and making informed choices are paramount. By researching potential supplements, prioritizing quality, tailoring choices to individual needs, and, most importantly, consulting with healthcare providers, seniors can safely and effectively use supplements to support their active lifestyles.

6

Staying Motivated and Making Informed Choices

In the journey toward a healthier lifestyle, seniors face unique challenges that can sometimes hinder their ability to maintain a nutritious diet. This chapter is dedicated to empowering older adults with the knowledge and strategies to stay motivated and make wise food choices. By understanding nutritional information and staying updated on the latest nutrition research, seniors can navigate their dietary needs with confidence and enthusiasm.

Reading Food Labels

Navigating the world of food labels is crucial for seniors aiming to make healthier dietary choices. Understanding the nutritional information on packaging can guide older adults in selecting foods that align with their health goals and dietary needs. This section explores critical aspects of food labels, offering insights into how to interpret them effectively.

Understanding the Nutrition Facts Panel

The Nutrition Facts panel on food packaging is a valuable resource for assessing the nutritional content of food items. Here's how to make the most of this information:

- **Serving Size:** Begin with the serving size and the number of servings per package. All the nutritional information listed refers to this amount, making it essential for portion control and understanding how much of each nutrient you consuming.
- **Calories:** The calorie count indicates the energy you'll get from one serving. Balancing calorie intake with expenditure is crucial for weight management, especially for seniors with lower energy needs.
- **Nutrients to Limit:** Pay special attention to saturated fats, trans fats, cholesterol, and sodium. Consuming less of these can help reduce the risk of chronic diseases. Look for foods with lower percentages of these nutrients.
- **Nutrients to Get More Of:** Dietary fiber, vitamins (A, C, D, E, and B vitamins), calcium, iron, magnesium, and potassium to support heart health, bone density, and overall well-being. Aim for foods higher in these nutrients.

Deciphering Ingredient Lists

Ingredients are listed in order of quantity, from highest to lowest. This can inform your choices in several ways:

- **Whole Foods First:** Products with whole foods (like whole grains, fruits, and vegetables) listed as the first ingredients are generally healthier.
- **Additives and Preservatives:** Be cautious of long lists of unfamiliar ingredients, indicating high levels of processed additives and

preservatives.

Interpreting Health Claims

Food packaging often includes health claims or certifications. While these can guide healthier choices, it's important to understand their meaning:

- **Health Claims:** Claims like "low sodium," "high fiber," or "no added sugars" are regulated and can help you choose products that fit your nutritional needs. However, reading the whole nutrition label is essential, as products may be low in one area but high in another (e.g., low in fat but high in sugar).
- **Certifications:** Labels such as "USDA Organic" or "Non-GMO Project Verified" provide information about farming practices and genetic modifications but don't necessarily indicate a product is healthier regarding nutritional content.

Staying Informed

For seniors committed to maintaining an active and healthy lifestyle, staying informed about the latest nutrition research and recommendations is very important. The field of nutrition science is continually evolving, with new findings that can impact dietary guidelines and influence our understanding of what constitutes a healthy diet. This section explores strategies for keeping in touch with these developments, ensuring seniors know to make informed dietary choices.

Leveraging Reputable Sources

Government Health Departments and Nutrition Organizations:

Websites of government health departments, such as the U.S. Department of Agriculture (USDA) and the National Institutes of Health (NIH), along with professional nutrition organizations, provide reliable, up-to-date information on nutrition guidelines and research. These resources often distill complex research findings into actionable dietary advice for the general public, including seniors.

Academic Journals and Publications: Academic journals offer a wealth of information for those interested in diving deeper into the science behind the guidelines. Accessing these may require more effort and a critical eye to interpret the data, but they provide insights directly from the researchers.

Consulting with Health Professionals

This is one thing that can't be stressed enough: consult with health professionals.

- **Regular Checkups with Healthcare Providers:** Incorporate discussions about nutrition into your regular checkups. Healthcare providers can offer advice tailored to your health status and may recommend adjustments to your diet based on the latest research findings.
- **Dietitians and Nutritionists:** Consulting with dietitians or nutritionists who are experts in the field of nutrition can provide personalized dietary guidance. They can translate the latest research into practical eating plans that meet your needs and health goals.

Continuous Learning

- **Workshops and Seminars:** Participating in workshops, seminars, or webinars focused on nutrition and health can be an excellent way to stay informed. These events often feature experts discussing the latest trends, research, and dietary recommendations.
- **Subscription to Health Newsletters:** Many reputable health organizations and nutrition experts offer newsletters summarizing the latest research and health news. Subscribing to these can provide regular updates right to your inbox.

Critical Evaluation of Information

- **Assess the Source:** When encountering new nutrition information, evaluate the source's credibility. Information from peer-reviewed scientific journals or reputable health organizations is more likely to be reliable than unverified online sources.
- **Beware of Fads and Quick Fixes:** Nutrition fads and diets promising quick fixes can be enticing, but they often need to be supported by scientific evidence. Be wary of claims that sound too good to be true, and always look for evidence-based information.

Seniors must constantly be acquainted and empowered to embrace healthy eating as a pleasurable and rewarding aspect of their lives. By developing strategies to overcome dietary challenges, enhancing their skills in reading food labels, and staying abreast of nutritional science, older adults can make informed choices that support their health and longevity.

7

Conclusion

This guide has navigated the essential aspects of nutrition for active seniors, emphasizing the importance of maintaining a balanced diet, understanding and supplementing nutritional gaps, and making informed food choices. We've dug into the significance of reading food labels, staying informed of the latest nutrition research and recommendations, and the critical role of consulting healthcare providers for personalized dietary advice.

The journey through nutrition for active seniors underscores a few key points:

- It is necessary to identify and address nutritional gaps with appropriate supplements, such as multivitamins, calcium, vitamin D, omega-3 fatty acids, and others, tailored to individual health needs and conditions.
- Be vigilant and informed when choosing supplements and foods, understand labels, and stay updated with nutritional science to ensure choices support overall health and well-being.
- The invaluable role of continuous learning and consultation with

healthcare professionals in adapting one's diet to meet changing health needs and leveraging the latest nutrition insights.

To all seniors striving for an active lifestyle, let this be a source of encouragement to embrace the journey of maintaining a nutritionally balanced diet. Your efforts to understand and apply the principles of good nutrition can significantly enhance your quality of life, enabling you to enjoy the activities you love with vigor and health. Remember, nutrition is a powerful tool in your arsenal for aging well; it supports not just physical health but mental and emotional well-being, too.

Embrace the challenge of staying informed, be proactive in making dietary choices, and don't hesitate to seek expert advice to tailor your nutrition plan to your unique needs. By doing so, you can ensure that your golden years are not just about living longer but better, fueled by the proper nutrients to keep you active, energized, and engaged in the joys of life. Let the healthy eating journey be a fulfilling part of your active lifestyle, enriching daily with vitality and well-being.

8

References

Kaloc, J., & Tereza. (2019, April 16). *Nutrition for active seniors – protein, carbs, and fat.* We Love Cycling Magazine. Retrieved March 26, 2024, from https://www.welovecycling.com/wide/2019/04/16/nutrition-for-active-seniors-protein-carbs-and-fat/

National Institute on Aging. (2021, January 2). *Vitamins and minerals for older adults.* Retrieved March 26, 2024, from https://www.nia.nih.gov/health/vitamins-and-supplements/vitamins-and-minerals-older-adults

National Institute on Aging. (2021, April 23). *Dietary supplements for older adults.* Retrieved March 26, 2024, from https://www.nia.nih.gov/health/vitamins-and-supplements/dietary-supplements-older-adults

Kernisan, L. (2023, June 15). *Q&A: How to Prevent, Detect, & Treat Dehydration in Aging Adults.* Better Health While Aging. Retrieved March 26, 2024, from https://betterhealthwhileaging.net/qa-how-to-prevent-diagnose-treat-dehydration-aging-adults/

National Institute on Aging. (2021, November 23). *Healthy meal planning: tips for older adults.* Retrieved March 26, 2024, from https://www.nia.nih.gov/health/healthy-eating-nutrition-and-diet/healthy-meal-planning-tips-older-adults

National Institute on Aging. (2022, February 22). *Healthy eating as you age: Know your food groups.* Retrieved March 26, 2024, from https://www.nia.nih.gov/health/healthy-eating-nutrition-and-diet/healthy-eating-you-age-know-your-food-groups

OpenAI. (2023). ChatGPT (GPT-4) [Software]. OpenAI. https://www.openai.com/